THE MAYR DIET COOKBOOK FOR BEGINNERS

A COMPLETE MAYR DIET WEIGHT LOSS PROGRAM GUIDE, LOTS OF DELICIOUS AND HEALTHY RECIPES.

DR AMANDA PATRICK

Copyright

Dr Amanda Patrick© Copyright 2021 – All rights reserved.

Except as permitted under the U.S. Copyright Act of 1976, the contents contained in this book may not be duplicated, reproduced, or transmitted without the prior written permission of the author or the publisher.

Under no circumstances will a legal responsibility or blame be directed towards the author or the publisher for any monetary loss, reparation, or damages based on the information in this book, directly or indirectly.

Disclaimer Notice:

Note that it is important that the following information contained in this book is for educational purposes only. After carrying out enough research work, we present a piece of detailed and accurate information as it relates to the present norm. We got the contents in this book from various sources, and hence, the intending readers are not given a warranty. We advise readers to talk to their licensed doctors before trying out the techniques given within this book.

By consenting to this document, the reader accepts that the author is not responsible for any loss either directly or indirectly that can be incurred as a result of the information contained within this book, and also the omissions, errors, or inadequacies of the reader.

Table of Contents

INTRODUCTION 6
WHAT IS THE MAYR METHOD DIET? 10
HOW THE MAYR METHOD DIET PLAN WORKS? 11
WHAT YOU SHOULD EXPECT WHEN ADOPTING THE MAYR METHOD DIET? 13
SECRETS TO THE MAYR METHOD DIET: 17
THE LIFESTYLE CHANGES WHICH ARE PART OF THE DIET? 21
IS THE MAYR METHOD DIET SAFE AND EFFECTIVE? 28
IS THE MAYR METHOD DIET RIGHT FOR YOU? 30
WHAT CAN YOU CONSUME ON THE MAYR METHOD DIET? 31
GUACAMOLE RECIPE 36
HEALTHY CHICKEN PAD THAI 38
SHRIMP WITH ZUCCHINI 42
HUMMUS PASTA 44
ZUCCHINI LASAGNA ROLL-UPS 46
ZUCCHINI FRITTERS WITH GARLIC HERB YOGURT SAUCE 48
WARM WHITE BEAN & KALE SALAD 53
CREAMY SHRIMP PASTA WITH CORN AND TOMATOES 55
TOMATO SPINACH CHICKEN SPAGHETTI 58
FENNEL SALAD WITH CUCUMBER AND DILL 62
SKINNY BANG BANG ZUCCHINI NOODLES 64
CHIMICHURRI SAUCE 67
LIGHTENED-UP CREAMY AVOCADO BASIL PESTO 69
CHICKEN LO MEIN 71
TACO CHICKEN SALAD 75
CAULIFLOWER KALE SOUP 77
CREAM OF ZUCCHINI SOUP 80
EASY SESAME QUINOA SALAD 82

SWEET POTATO BRUSSELS SPROUT QUINOA BOWL	85
CURRIED CAULIFLOWER	87
ITALIAN FENNEL AND ORANGE SALAD	89
MAPLE SRIRACHA ROASTED CAULIFLOWER	91
BAKED CINNAMON APPLE CHIPS	93
ZUCCHINI NOODLES WITH AVOCADO SAUCE	95
ROASTED BROCCOLI WITH ASIAGO, GARLIC AND ALMONDS	98
ROASTED CHICKEN THIGHS WITH FENNEL & LEMON	101
SHAVED FENNEL WHITE BEAN SALAD WITH OLIVE VINAIGRETTE	104
SPIRALIZED CARROT AND FENNEL SALAD	107
CABBAGE SALAD WITH CORN	109
SPINACH AND SUN-DRIED TOMATO ZOODLES	111
CLASSIC POTATO PANCAKES	115
EASY CREAMY CHICKEN PICCATA	117
SWEET AND SOUR CUCUMBER NOODLES	120
ROASTED BROCCOLI QUINOA SALAD	122
HONEY GARLIC ROASTED CARROTS	124
KALE SALAD	126
GARLIC HERB ROASTED POTATOES CARROTS AND GREEN BEANS	128
ROASTED CAULIFLOWER STEAKS	130
HOT TURKEY AND CHEESE PARTY ROLLS	133
ROASTED BROCCOLI FENNEL SOUP	135
LEEK, SWEET POTATO AND ROSEMARY SOUP	138
CREAMY ASPARAGUS AND LEEK SOUP	141
WILD SALMON WITH BRAISED VEGETABLES	143
GRILLED BEET AND FENNEL SALAD	146
CABBAGE, CUCUMBER AND FENNEL SALAD WITH DILL	149
CORN SOUP WITH LEMONGRASS	152
RED BEET CAKE	154

RACK OF LAMB WITH POLENTA...156
CONCLUSION 158

Introduction

Are you up for some weight loss, but you don't know how? In the past, you may have attempted to lose weight on other diets, but no matter how hard you tried, you realized that either you regained weight or you never lost weight in the first place. If they have become too difficult to comply with or are not intended to be long-term weight loss strategies, all of these choices are just not good for you. However, just because some diet that promised instant results didn't turn out doesn't mean you're stuck at whatever weight you're currently at. You can lose weight, and you can do so in a way that is safe and healthy and without leaving out all the foods you might enjoy.

You may have learned about the Mayr Method diet if you want to lose weight, but you wonder if this kind of weight loss plan is healthy and successful. We've found a proven way to help you lose weight and get healthier while this will direct you to learn more about Mayr Method and whether it's right for you to help you reach goals of wellness, fitness, and weight loss!

"Believe it or not, according to VivaMayr workers, the Mayr Method has been around for more than a century, based on the "Mayr Cure" developed by Franz Xaver Mayr in Austria in the 1920s, also known as F.X. Mayr. The program's fundamentals have to do with a "clean" gut and an emphasis on eating food that massages the digestive systems. Maximilian Schubert, VivaMayr's medical director told NBC's Today that the Mayr diet has rarely changed over time: "The main idea behind this if people have a healthy gut system and healthy digestive system, then they are going to have a holistic approach of health," Schubert said.

People are usually first introduced to this diet by visiting VivaMayr or one of its many wellness retreats around the world during a prolonged stay and a series of consultations. This method combines modern complementary medicine with traditional diagnostics and therapies. As soon as one's condition is treated, proper nutrition combined with exercise & improved mental awareness become the building blocks of your new life.

The first guidance made to many clients is to start a new fasting schedule. In general, the first step in all occasions is a monotone & restricted diet, to really calm down the body system, food-wise. In addition to a short-term fast, the program will also involve a prescribed cleanse, taking new or expanded vitamins & supplements in which is regarded as "detoxification process."

In addition to specifying a fasting schedule, dieters will also avoid consuming sugar or drinking coffee (anything containing caffeine) and alcohol during the program. Quite often, people will have some headaches & mood changes in the first 3 or 4 days — afterwards, they recover very well again.

This is The Mayr Diet's comprehensive review, detailing what you need to understand.

What is the Mayr Method Diet?

The Mayr Diet, also known as the Viva Mayr Diet, is based on the Mayr Cure, developed 100 years ago by the Austrian physician Franz Xaver Mayr, MD.

Although adopting the Mayr Method program, some celebrities, including Rebel Wilson, have effectively lost weight.

It's focused on the idea that individuals with ordinary eating habits and foods poison their digestive systems. The Mayr Method plan integrates traditional therapies with complementary medicine to address health conditions if they occur, and to boost mental awareness by using exercise plus good nutrition. The founders of the Mayr Method tout a flatter stomach, more muscle, and radiant skin.

How The Mayr Method Diet Plan Works?

The philosophy of the diet focuses on eating well and making your digestive health an important part of your overall health. It works to get followers to avoid snacking, decrease their consumption of gluten and milk, and even chew their foods longer.

It all starts out with a detox of sugar and caffeine. It also touches on certain improvements in lifestyles, such as concentrating 40 to 60 times on chewing every bite. Talking, or looking at your phone, reading while you eat are prohibited (the aim is to get you to chew slowly and be more conscious of your food). Meals contain high-alkaline, whole foods, such as vegetables and fish.

Schubert suggests starting with some moderate fasting if you're looking to get started at home. "In general, the first step on all occasions is a monotone and restricted diet, to really calm down the body system, food-wise," he explained.

"This diet also requires cleansing and consuming vitamins or supplements to reduce side effects associated with what Schubert called the "detoxification process." Headaches, nausea, stomach cramps and fatigue were potential side effects.

"Quite often, clients will still have some headaches & mood changes in the first 3 or 4 days. Afterwards, they recover very well again," Schubert explains.

What You Should Expect When Adopting the Mayr Method Diet?

You concentrate on enhancing the gut and general health and wellbeing while adopting the Mayr Method diet for weight loss.

These are the main components of this weight loss diet:

- Nutrition and gut health
- Exercise
- Medication
- Awareness

Nutrition and Gut Health

When using the Mayr Approach for weight loss, use the following nutritional recommendations:

Dieters are instructed to:

- Start the program with sugar and caffeine detox
- Quit snacking
- Making breakfast part of the routine, dropping dinner potentially.
- Refrain from consuming raw foods in the evening after 4 p.m.
- Decrease consumption of dairy foods
- Reduce intake of gluten-containing foods, such as wheat, barley & rye food products
- Chew foods for a longer period (chew each bite of food 40 to 60 times)
- Consume high-alkaline whole foods like fruits, vegetables, tofu, nuts, seeds, legumes, and fish
- Do away from highly processed foods
- Concentrate on mindfulness while consuming.

The bottom line is that by adopting the Mayr Method diet, you will consume mostly organic, whole foods and eat less calories overall.

Exercise

The Mayr Method weight loss plan has more to offer than just modifying your eating habits. In addition to eating nutritious foods, you'll exercise daily, up to 6 days each week. To achieve optimum performance, combine physical workouts with resistance training.

Medicine

Getting the right medical care for risk factors for chronic diseases will dramatically reduce the chance of developing a condition that is debilitating, such as diabetes, heart disease, or cancer.

In addition to making healthy lifestyle improvements, visit the doctor periodically to better regulate your blood pressure, cholesterol, or triglycerides, with medical care if necessary.

If your doctor suggests that you take chronic disease drugs, when you continue to lose weight, you may be able to decrease your dosage or remove the need for medications entirely.

Awareness

Concentrate on the task at hand each time you consume food to avoid getting distracted and consuming too many calories overall. Watching television, playing with your phone, reading, & chatting on the phone or with friends can be common distractions.

Secrets To The Mayr Method Diet:

Eat Alkaline Foods

Naturally, many whole, minimally processed foods such as fruit, vegetables, legumes, and nuts are more alkaline, which is why it is a good idea to consume alkaline foods while selecting the Mayr Method diet.

You don't just have to eat alkaline foods, however, because if you're in good health, your body can handle pH levels on its own properly.

Chew Each Bite of Food 40-60 Times

It's boring and time-consuming to chew each bite of food 40-60 times, and not realistic in any case. This technique, however, could help you eat slowly and consume less calories overall, which is helpful as you strive to reach your target weight.

Nix Sugar and Caffeine

Removing sugar is an excellent technique for healthy eating, but reducing caffeine will drain your energy when you're used to drinking coffee or tea. In reality, studies show that caffeine can improve your metabolism, help reduce body mass index (BMI) and body fat, and aid in weight loss. However, avoid caffeinated sodas because they contain added sugar that can lead to excessive weight gain.

Avoid Snacks

One way to reduce the general calorie intake for weight loss is to avoid snacks, as long as you don't overindulge at mealtime. To effectively lose weight, however, you don't have to ignore snacks completely.

In fact, in some cases, not consuming snacks can lead to between-meal exhaustion or overindulging at mealtime.

Consume either a small meal or a snack every few hours or so.

Reduce Dairy Foods

As recommended by the founders of the Mayr Method diet plan, reducing your consumption of dairy foods is not sufficient to shed excess weight. Low-fat dairy foods such as Greek yogurt, low-fat cottage cheese, and low-fat milk actually provide you with high-quality protein, calcium, and vitamin D that your body requires to work properly.

Research indicates that in women seeking to lose weight, consuming calcium-rich dairy foods tends to improve weight loss and improve body composition. Therefore, nixing dairy foods is not necessary, but instead select calcium-fortified plant milks or yoghurts if you choose to avoid them.

Avoid Gluten

For weight loss, avoiding foods with gluten is not important either, but if you have Celiac disease or gluten sensitivity, you can avoid wheat, barley, and rye items. Steer clear of heavily processed foods containing gluten, such as white bread.

Practice Mindfulness

Using mindfulness is also an effective weight loss approach, as recommended by the founders of the Mayr Method diet. Although you don't have to chew your food a certain amount of times to absorb less calories, a successful weight loss approach is to eat slowly. That you don't get distracted when consuming.

The Lifestyle Changes Which Are Part Of The Diet?

This diet method also focuses extensively on the lifestyle and attitudes through meals. One big feature is chewing a piece of food about 40 and 60 times before swallowing, and Schubert said at VivaMayr that workers use chewing trainers to get people used to the activity, a piece of slightly stale bread.

Kirkpatrick said there is some evidence that indicates that repeatedly chewing a single bite will help with weight loss.

It is more intuitive eating approach, where you're being more mindful, where you're really kind of taking an extra step to number one appreciate food, but number two, to kind of slow down the rate of eating.

Other habits repeated in the Mayr diet include, "stopping when you are satisfied, drinking between meals & not with meals, (and) not consuming after 4 or 5 p.m. according to Schubert. He also said that leaving "four to five hours" between meals is necessary so that you can "fully digest" your food.

The importance of exercise in the diet was also emphasised by Schubert. "Without exercise, you can't reach any health goal," he said.

When adopting this form of well-balanced, safe weight loss lifestyle plan, expect:

Eat a Variety of Healthy Foods

A wide variety of nutritious foods to be consumed, such as:

- Non-starchy vegetables

- Fruits
- Peas, beans, lentils, and other legumes
- Whole grains
- Avocados, olives, olive oil & other heart-healthy fats
- Starchy vegetables
- Nuts and seeds
- Fish, chicken, eggs, tofu & other protein food

Get Motivational Support

It is always half the fight to stay motivated for weight loss, as your emotions will get in the way of obtaining your ideal weight.

See a doctor regarding potential mental health therapies that can relax you or lift your mood and level of motivation during weight loss if you suffer from chronic stress, anxiety or depression that influences eating habits and your calorie intake.

Fat-Burning Workouts

Changing your diet is not the only essential part of getting safe and lean and remaining healthy. For reaching your target weight and keeping it for life, daily exercise is important. You can maximize the benefits of healthier eating improvements if you make time for at least 30 minutes of exercise everyday. In addition, aim to keep moving all through the day, not just during workouts.

Aim to accomplish at least 45 minutes of everyday activities, such as housework, outdoor yard work, grocery shopping, cooking, or walking the dog, that keep your body in motion.

Take Dietary Supplements

During weight loss, the usefulness of taking dietary supplements is two-fold. Supplements will decrease the risk of nutritional deficiencies in vitamins, minerals and other substances and increase energy levels.

Some women's weight loss supplements, such as protein bars, protein drinks, and fiber supplements, help improve satiety, making it easier to consume less weight loss calories.

Set Goals

One of the easiest ways to achieve the bodyweight you want is to set targets. In contrast to not setting goals, studies indicate that target setting contributes to greater long-term weight loss. Pick goals for weekly weigh-ins, waist circumference, completed workout minutes, sleep hours, and goals for diet.

Target to lose between 1-2 pounds per week to drop weight at a healthy, productive pace and reach a lifetime target weight you can sustain.

Set targets to avoid sugar drinks, candy, fried foods, refined grains, alcoholic drinks, highly processed foods, and many fast foods. Every now and then, you may give yourself a cheat day, but avoid junk food as much as possible.

Self-Monitor

Self-monitor parameters for health and wellness and keep track of the improvement of weight loss along your journey. To hold yourself accountable for meeting the goals you set for yourself, log your food consumption, minutes of exercise, hours of sleep, body weight, and more in a journal. Studies suggest that daily weigh-ins are more efficient than checking in less often for weight loss.

Listen to Your Body

It's essential to listen to your body when it comes to nutrition, exercise, sleep, and overall health and wellness.

Eat a healthy snack or meal if you feel hungry, and quit eating when you feel full. When you need more of these vital nutrients, your body might crave foods rich in vitamin C, such as citrus fruits, or protein-rich foods such as chicken, fish, eggs, or tofu.

Is The Mayr Method Diet Safe And Effective?

This way of eating can all be healthy and effective as long as you don't severely limit calories or foods while following the Mayr Method diet.

If you try the Mayr Method Diet at home, you can concentrate on a few takeaways, including tips to eat more carefully at mealtimes. Most people rush their meals and don't chew our food enough, and chewing is important to ensure proper digestion and maximum absorption later on in our digestive tract, adding that somewhere between 30 to 40 chews per mouthful is something you should aim for. It requires around 20 minutes for your body to signify the brain that it is full. If we are consuming too quickly, we can easily overeat before our brain is able to signal we are full.

Seeking supplements to imitate any clinic procedure is one thing you shouldn't do at home. "If you see [any product] with detox or cleanse slapped on it, be suspicious and ask questions. For gut health in particular, staying hydrated & incorporating probiotic-rich foods such as kefir, kombucha and yogurt into your diet is acceptable. Food first before reaching for a pill or supplement.

Is The Mayr Method Diet Right For You?

Although success has been promoted by Rebel Wilson and other celebrities while adopting Mayr Method meal plans, the diet is not for all. If too restrictive to your preference, know that you have extra, well-balanced choices.

Many of the concepts used in the Mayr Method plan are components worthy of implementation regardless of the body weight and health goals, such as consuming whole foods, eliminating added sugar, having daily exercise, and practicing mindfulness when eating.

What Can You Consume On The Mayr Method Diet?

Creating your own meals according to suggested menu plans is perfectly appropriate, although you may want to try them for a few days first.

Ultimately, the diet is also said to be based on the fundamentals of an alkaline diet, but Stefani Sassos, MS, RD, CDN, the registered dietitian of the Good Housekeeping Institute, states that the foods on the shopping list of the diet plan are not necessarily found in true alkaline-forward diets. Lots of food on this list, including polenta, risotto, meat & dairy aren't normally allowed on an alkaline diet as they are thought to be 'acidic.'" In the end, though, it does not matter, explains Sassos, because the advantages of the alkaline diet have to do with consuming more fruits, decreasing the consumption of sugar and refined foods, and drinking more water (all items you can do without recommending a diet!).

The Mayr Method Diet shopping list is as follows:

Dairy:

Butter, organic eggs, goat cheese, sour cream, Parmesan cheese, cottage cheese, rice milk, oat milk.

Proteins:

Smoked trout, trout fillet, skinless turkey breast, lamb loin, salmon fillets, smoked salmon, beef fillets, organic silken tofu, and char caviar.

Grains:

Buckwheat flour, ground oats (and other ingredients to make your own bread), corn flakes, millet, spelt flour, polenta, risotto rice.

Nuts and seeds:

Walnuts, sesame seeds, amaranth seeds, and almonds.

Fruits:

Olives, raisins, apricots, prunes, apples, berries, pomegranates, oranges, citrus fruit, bananas, papaya, mangoes, avocados.

Vegetables:

Onions, spinach, radishes, celery, carrots, fennel, potatoes, kohlrabi, vine tomatoes, lettuce, sprouts, broccoli, turnips, and chickpeas.

Beverages:

Green tea, pomegranate juice, and water.

Condiments & seasonings:

Vegetable stock, stevia, rock salt, extra-virgin olive oil, cold-pressed oils (including linseed, hemp, and walnut), coconut oil, balsamic vinegar, honey, maple syrup, cider vinegar, cream of tartar, soya sauce.

Some delicious Mayr Diet Recipes are below

Enjoy, Lose weight and Stay Healthy!

Guacamole Recipe

Recipes:

- 1/4 cup of finely minced onion
- Three ripe Haas of avocados
- 1 1/2 tablespoons of fresh lime juice (or lemon juice)
- One big Plum or Roma tomato, deseeded & diced
- 1/4 cup of cilantro leaves & tender stems, chopped
- 1/2 teaspoon of ground cumin, optional
- 1/2 teaspoon of salt, or more
- 1 to 2 teaspoons of minced jalapeño or serrano pepper, with seeds & membrane removed, non-compulsory

Directions

1. In a small clean bowl, add the diced onion, then cover with warm water, set aside for 5 minutes, and

drain. The onions are "de-flamed" by this, making them less intense.

2. Gently cut the avocados into half, & remove the pit lengthwise. Scoop the flesh out, then add it to a bowl.

3. Use a clean fork to mash until creamy but still chunky, then add lime juice. Tomatoes, cilantro, cumin, drained de-flamed onions, salt, and diced peppers are mixed together (if using).

1. Taste and adjust the guacamole with added salt, pepper, or lime juice. By moving the plastic wrap down onto the guacamole, serve immediately or cover with plastic wrap and refrigerate up to one day.

Healthy Chicken Pad Thai

Recipes:

- 5 oz of brown rice noodles
- Two tablespoons of olive oil
- 1 lb of chicken breasts pounded thinly
- 1 cup of red peppers sliced into thin pieces
- 2 cups of carrots sliced into thin pieces
- 1/2 cup of chopped onion
- One tablespoon of garlic minced
- 1 cup of Bean sprouts
- Two large eggs

For the Sauce:

- One tablespoon peanut butter
- Two tablespoons honey
- Two tablespoons lime juice
- 1.5 tablespoons rice wine vinegar

- ¼ cup of fish sauce
- ¼ cup of coconut aminos or a low sodium soy sauce

For Garnish:

- 1/4 cup green onions sliced thinly
- ⅓ cup peanuts crushed or chopped
- red pepper flakes (optional)
- lime wedges (optional)
- cilantro (optional)

Directions

1. Cut the chicken into square 1-inch pieces. Gently heat the olive oil in a big clean pan over medium-high heat. Add the cubed chicken to the pan and cook for 12-15 minutes over medium-high heat until fully browned and cooked!

2. Carry a clean pot of water to a boil during chicken cooking + cook rice noodles according to the instructions on the package.
3. While cooking noodles/chicken, whisk the ingredients for the sauce together and set off to the side. Chop the veggies.
4. Detach the chicken from the pan + put it aside in a large bowl once the chicken has cooked. Try to leave the pan with the oil.
5. Add the peppers, carrots, garlic, and onion to the oil and sauté for 10 minutes, uncovered. Stir in the bean sprouts after ten minutes and cook for an additional two minutes.
6. Push vegetables into the pan on one side of the pan + crack eggs. Scramble for about two minutes until the eggs are cooked.

7. Stir veggie/egg mixture together. Take it out of the pan and set it aside with the chicken.

8. Add the mixture of sauce to the empty pan (you don't need to clean the pan!) & bring to a low boil whilst constantly stirring for one minute. It should bubble and thicken the sauce slightly.

9. In the saucepan, add the cooked veggies, cooked chicken, and cooked noodles and toss to combine.

10. Garnish well with peanuts. Optional garnish: lime, green onions, cilantro.

Shrimp With Zucchini

Recipes:

- 2 tbsp. Of olive oil
- 450 gr. Of shrimp, peeled and deveined
- Three minced garlic cloves.
- 1/2 tsp. of chopped red pepper
- 2 tbsp. of lemon juice
- 1/2 tsp. of lemon zest
- 1/2 teaspoon of salt
- 1/4 tsp of ground black pepper
- Three medium zucchinis, spiralized
- 2 tbsp of grated Parmesan
- Two tablespoons of chopped parsley

Directions

1. Carefully Heat a skillet over medium-high heat using oil.

2. Then proceed to Add the shrimp, black pepper, sea salt, & red pepper.
3. Proceed to cook until shrimp are pink, for up to five minutes.
4. Add the lemon zest, lemon juice & garlic.
5. Add the spiralized zucchini noodles & Parmesan, and mix very well.
6. It can also be garnished with parsley for a lovely decoration!

Hummus Pasta

Recipes:

- Two tablespoons olive oil
- One medium onion sliced
- Two garlic cloves sliced
- 1 cup spinach
- 1 cup plain hummus
- 1 pound spaghetti pasta
- Juice of 1 lemon + zest
- ¼ cup of freshly chopped basil plus more for serving
- Pinch of crushed red pepper

Directions

1. Over high heat, bring a large pot of salted water to a low boil. Add the pasta & cook following the package instructions until al dente. Move aside one cup of

pasta cooking water, then drain the pasta and put it back in the pot to keep warm.
2. Gently heat the olive oil in a clean big skillet over medium heat. Add the onions and cook for 5-7 minutes or until they are soft and fragrant. Add the garlic & cook until fragrant or for 30 seconds. Add the spinach & cook until it is slightly wilted, or 1 minute.
3. Add the hummus, ½ cup of pasta cooking water, lemon juice, and lemon zest, and stir until the sauce is creamy. Put extra pasta water, as needed, to thin the sauce a bit at a time.
4. Transfer to the skillet the cooked pasta, turn off the heat, and toss it all together. Add basil and crushed red pepper to top.
5. If desired, serve immediately with parmesan cheese or basil.

Zucchini Lasagna Roll-Ups

Recipes:

- Six big zucchinis
- 1 (16-oz.) container of ricotta
- 3/4 c. freshly grated Parmesan, divided
- Two big eggs
- 1/2 tsp. of garlic powder
- Kosher salt
- Freshly ground pepper (black)
- 1 cup of marinara
- 1 cup of grated mozzarella

Directions

1. Preheat the oven to 400 degrees. Lengthwise slice zucchini into 1/8 inches thick strips, then place strips on a baking sheet lined with a paper towel to drain.

2. Make a mixture of ricotta: combine ricotta, 1/2 cup Parmesan cheese, eggs, and garlic powder in a small bowl, and season well with salt & pepper.

3. Spread a thin layer of marinara on the bottom of a 9-inch by 13-inch baking dish. Spoon a thin layer of sauce on both slices of zucchini, spread the ricotta mixture on top, and sprinkle with mozzarella. Roll up and place in a tightly packed baking dish.

4. Sprinkle with another 1/4 cup of Parmesan cheese. Bake for up to 20 minutes, until the zucchini is tender and the cheese melts.

Zucchini Fritters With Garlic Herb Yogurt Sauce

Recipes:

Garlic Herb Yogurt Sauce:

- 1/2 cup of plain Greek or regular yogurt
- Two teaspoons of chopped parsley
- 1 Tablespoon of chopped fresh mint
- 2 Tablespoons of fresh lemon juice
- 1 Tablespoon of olive oil
- One teaspoon of honey
- One heaping teaspoon of minced garlic
- salt & fresh ground black pepper, to taste

Fritters:

- 2 cups of shredded zucchini (2 small or one large zucchini)
- 1 cup of shredded sweet potato (1 small, peeled)

- 1/3 cup of finely chopped onion
- 1 and 1/2 teaspoons of salt
- Two big eggs
- One heaping teaspoon of minced garlic
- 2 Tablespoons of chopped parsley
- 2 Tablespoons of chopped fresh mint
- 1/2 teaspoon of freshly ground pepper black
- 1/3 cup of cornmeal
- 1 Tablespoon of cornstarch
- 1/3 cup of olive oil

Directions

1. Create the yogurt sauce by whisking together all the ingredients for the yogurt sauce except the salt and pepper. Taste to taste, then add salt/pepper to taste. Cover and refrigerate until ready to serve.

2. Make the fritters: In a large strainer, place the shredded zucchini, sweet potato, and onion. Put one teaspoon of salt on top and mix it with a large wooden spoon. To start draining some of the water out of the vegetables, press down with your hands. Let it sit for some time in the sink.

3. Meanwhile, with paper towels or a clean dish towel, line a large bowl (easier to use a towel!). Place the mixture of vegetables in the bowl and top the dish towel with more paper towels or fold over. Start pressing down; you need as much liquid as possible to get out.

4. As required, grab more paper towels or a new dish towel. Note: you can also simply wring the vegetables over the sink in the dishtowel. Simply keep, wringing! Let the vegetables sit for 45 minutes on the towels, then press again. The goal is to

remove as much moisture as possible. Otherwise, they'll be soggy fritters. How much water you wring out will amaze you!

5. In a large bowl, whisk the eggs together. Whisk in the garlic, parsley, mint, remaining 1/2 teaspoon salt, and pepper beat. Fold in the vegetables and add the cornmeal and cornstarch until all is mixed together.

6. Heat oil over medium-high heat in a skillet. Use a fork to scoop up about two tablespoons of the zucchini mixture when hot (I always eyeball the amount). The bottom of the bowl may have liquid pooling, so make sure you use a fork, so the excess liquid is not in your fritter.

7. Top the hot skillet with the mixture and flatten it with a spatula. Repeat with a few more, making sure the skillet does not overcrowd. Cook until golden

brown, each side for about 3 minutes. Transfer until finished to a paper towel-lined plate.

8. Serve warm fritters and sauce with yogurt.

Warm White Bean & Kale Salad

Recipes:

- Four slices of sourdough bread

- Olive oil

- Haven's Kitchen Herby Chimichurri

- One bunch of dinosaur kale, chopped

- Two 15oz cans of white beans, drained & rinsed

- ½ of red onion, thinly sliced

Directions

1. Make croutons: gently heat the oven to 400 degrees F. Have the bread cut into cubes. Toss the olive oil with a glug. Spread on a clean baking sheet and bake until crispy, for about 10 minutes. Remove from the oven and toss the croutons in a bowl with about half the Chimichurri pouch. Just set aside.

2. Heat enough oil in a clean large skillet to coat the pan. Add the kale, and add the beans and the red onion when you see it start to wilt.

3. Cut the heat and squeeze another ¼ pouch of Chimichurri in the pan once they're warm and stir. Toss to taste with croutons, more sauce, and salt.

Creamy Shrimp Pasta With Corn And Tomatoes

Recipes:

- 8 ounces of linguine, spaghetti, or similar
- 1/2 cup of reserved pasta water
- Two tablespoons of butter, divided
- 1 lb. of shrimp, peeled & deveined (tail off or on, it's up to you)
- One teaspoon of salt, divided
- 1–2 cloves of garlic, minced
- 2 cups of cherry tomatoes, halved
- 2–3 ears of cooked or grilled fresh sweet corn, kernels cut off the cob
- 1 cup of fresh spinach, chopped
- a squeeze of lemon juice
- 1/2 - 3/4 cup of heavy cream

- fresh basil or Parmesan for topping
- salt & pepper to taste

Directions

1. Cook pasta according to the directions for the package. Drain, toss with oil, and set aside to prevent sticking.

2. Over medium heat, gently heat a large non-stick skillet. To the pan, add 1 tablespoon of butter. Sprinkle with 1/2 teaspoon salt and add the shrimp. Flip & cook until the shrimp is cooked. To keep warm, set aside and cover.

3. Add the garlic and one tablespoon of the remaining butter. Add the corn and tomatoes; sauté for 1-2 minutes. Spinach added; sauté until wilted.

4. Add the shrimp to the pan again. Add the remaining half of a teaspoon of salt and lemon juice. Add the cream and bring it to a low boil.
5. Toss your sauce with the cooked pasta. As needed, add the reserved pasta water. Top with basil, Parmesan, salt, or black pepper, which is freshly cracked.

Tomato Spinach Chicken Spaghetti

Recipes:

- 1/4 cup of sun-dried tomatoes chopped, drained of oil
- Two tablespoons of olive oil drained from sun-dried tomatoes
- 1/2 lb of chicken boneless and skinless (preferably, boneless skinless thighs), chopped
- 1/4 teaspoon of salt
- 1/4 teaspoon of red pepper flakes
- 1/4 teaspoon of salt
- Four Roma tomatoes chopped
- 1/4 cup fresh basil leaves chopped
- 8 oz of spinach fresh
- Three garlic cloves chopped
- 8 oz of spaghetti pasta

- Three tablespoons of olive oil (use high-quality olive oil or oil from the sun-dried tomatoes jar)

Directions

1. On medium-low heat, add the chopped sun-dried tomatoes and two tablespoons of the olive oil drained from the sun-dried tomatoes to a clean large skillet.
2. Add a chicken chopped. I have used and prefer to use boneless skinless chicken thighs, but you can also use chopped chicken breast.
3. Add red pepper flakes & salt over all of the ingredients in the clean skillet.
4. Gently cook on medium heat until the chicken is cooked through & no longer pink, about up to five minutes.

5. Top the chicken skillet with chopped tomatoes, chopped fresh basil leaves, fresh spinach, and chopped garlic. Cook for about 3-5 minutes on a medium heat until the spinach wilts a little, and the tomatoes release some of their juices. Withdraw from the heat.

6. Taste, and, if required, add more salt to taste. Cover the lid and keep the heat off.

7. According to package instructions, cook pasta until al dente.

8. Drain the skillet with the chicken and vegetables and add the cooked and drained pasta.

9. Reheat on low heat, mix well, add more seasonings, if desired (salt and pepper). Withdraw from the heat.

10. At this point in time, when the vegetables & pasta are off heat, you can proceed to add more olive oil. It's voluntary but very tasty!

Fennel Salad With Cucumber And Dill

Recipes:

- Two big fennel bulbs- trimmed and cored
- Three small Persian cucumbers
- 1/2 cup of fresh chopped dill
- 1/4 cup of white onion, thinly sliced (optional)
- ⅓ cup of olive oil
- Three tablespoons of lemon juice (Meyer lemon is nice, or sherry vinegar or, champagne, or red wine vinegar)
- pepper to taste
- kosher salt to taste

Directions

1. Halve the fennel bulbs and remove the hard core from them.

2. Shave the fennel thinly using a mandolin and place it in a bowl (Or finely slice as thin as possible).
3. Finely slice the mandolin with the cucumber and chop the dill. Slice onion finely.
4. Add the olive oil, lemon, salt, and cracked pepper and place everything in a bowl. Before serving, leave to marinate in the fridge for 15 minutes.
5. Taste, adjust the lemon and salt.

Skinny Bang Bang Zucchini Noodles

Course: Main Dishes

Preparation Time: 10 Minutes

Cook Time: 10 Minutes

Total Time: 20 Minutes

Yields: 4 Servings

Recipes:

- One tablespoon of olive oil
- Four medium zucchini (spiralized)

For the Sauce:

- 1/4 cup plus two tablespoons of light mayonnaise
- 1/4 cup plus two tablespoons of fat-free plain Greek yoghurt
- One and a half tablespoons of honey

- Two teaspoons of lime juice
- 1/4 cup plus two tablespoons of Thai sweet chilli sauce
- One and a half teaspoon of sriracha sauce

Directions

1. Firstly, you should cook any proteins on the stove, if that is what you are using and put aside.

To Cook The Zucchini:

2. Gently add olive oil to a large clean skillet and then bring from medium to high heat. Add in zucchini noodles, as soon as the oil is hot. Continue with the cooking until water discharges and zucchini are just cooked (tender but still crisp). Put off the heat.
3. Now, you should drain the zucchini noodles and then allow the noodles to rest for around ten minutes and drain again any water discharged.

4. In a large clean container, Mix with a whisk all sauce recipes, until it gets smooth. Taste and adjust if required.

5. Gently pour the sauce into four small clean containers. Now, mix in zucchini noodles with the proteins too and then add to meal prep containers as soon as it is entirely cooled. Keep in a refrigerator & eat within 3 days.

Note

Drain any water that may be discharged from the noodles. Toss in the sauce.

Chimichurri Sauce

Preparation Time: 5 Minutes

Total Time: 5 Minutes

Yields: One And A Half Cup

Recipes:

- One bunch of worth cilantro leaves (few stems)
- One bunch of worth parsley leaves (few stems)
- 1/4 cup of red wine vinegar
- 3/4 cup of olive oil
- Half teaspoon of Pepper
- One teaspoon of red pepper flakes (if desired)
- Three cloves of garlic
- Half teaspoon of salt

Directions:

1. Firstly, you should combine all the recipes in a clean food processor. Now pulse for around thirty to forty-five seconds until it is well combined.
2. Proceed to serve on cooked seafood, meat and vegetables.

Note

You can store leftovers a clean airtight bowl or pint mason jar refrigerated for fourteen days or frozen for six months.

Lightened-Up Creamy Avocado Basil Pesto

Preparation Time: 10 Minutes

Total Time: 10 Minutes

Yields: 4 Servings (1 cup each)

Recipes:

- Half large ripe avocado
- One cup of packed fresh basil leaves
- Two tablespoons of pine nuts
- Two cloves of garlic
- Three tablespoons water (plus extra if required)
- One tablespoon of fresh lemon juice
- Sea salt (as required)
- 1/4 cup of grated Parmesan cheese

Directions

1. Firstly, Add avocado, basil, pine nuts, lemon juice and garlic to a clean food processor and then pulse for twenty seconds or until the pesto are well chopped. Add in water and process once more until totally smooth (you can add more water if required). Transfer to a clean container and then gently stir in the cheese.
2. You can keep in a sealed mason jar or a clean airtight bowl and then refrigerate.

Note

Pesto is best if used within a few days; else you can freeze it for some months.

Chicken Lo Mein

Preparation Time: 15 Minutes

Cook Time: 15 Minutes

Total Time: 30 Minutes

Yields: 6 Servings

Recipes:

- Three green onions (chopped)
- 16 ounces ramen noodles (or any other Asian style noodles)

For the Sauce:

- Two tablespoons of soy sauce low sodium
- One tablespoon of brown sugar packed
- One tablespoon of oyster sauce
- Two tablespoons of dark soy sauce

- One teaspoon of sesame oil
- One teaspoon of ground black pepper
- One teaspoon of hoisin sauce

For the Chicken:

- Two tablespoons of soy sauce
- Two tablespoons of olive oil
- One-pound chicken breasts skinless and boneless, cut into small pieces
- Three cloves of garlic minced
- One teaspoon of fresh ginger minced

For the Veggies:

- Two cups of shiitake mushrooms sliced
- Two tablespoons of olive oil
- One large onion (chopped)
- One cup of Chinese cabbage (shredded)

- One cup of carrots julienned

Directions:

1. Firstly, you should cook the noodles following the package directions. Drain and put aside.
2. In a small clean container whisk all the sauce recipes together, then put aside.
3. In another medium-sized clean container toss together the chicken with the ginger, garlic and soy sauce.
4. Proceed to heat the olive oil well in a big clean wok. Add the chicken as soon as it is hot. Add the seasoned chicken and cook for approximately five minutes or until the chicken begins to appear brown and isn't pink inside anymore. Move chicken to a clean plate and put aside.

5. Add the other two tablespoons of olive oil to the wok and then add the cabbage, shiitake mushrooms, onion and carrots to the wok. Cook for one minute and keep tossing around.
6. Now add the chicken to the wok once again. Add the prepared sauce, cooked noodles and toss all together.
7. Put off the heat.
8. You should garnish with green onions and then serve to enjoy.

Taco Chicken Salad

Preparation Time: 15 Minutes

Total Time: 15 Minutes

Yield: 6 Servings

Recipes:

- Half cup of mayo, or to taste
- Three to four cups of cooked chicken (diced)
- Half red pepper (diced)
- Half green pepper (diced)
- Half medium tomato (diced)
- Half cup red onion (diced)
- One tablespoon of chilli powder
- 1/4 teaspoon of chipotle powder
- Half cup chopped cilantro
- 1/4 tablespoon of paprika

- Half lime juice

- Half tablespoon of garlic powder

- Half teaspoon of cumin

- 1/4 teaspoon of cayenne

Directions

1. In a big clean container, mix mayo with the spices first to equally combine.
2. Add in vegetables and chicken, mix well to evenly coat with seasoned mayo.
3. Gently squeeze in lime juice over chicken salad and mix once more to combine.
4. You can top with whatever garnishes you desire (diced green onion, more cilantro). You can store in the fridge in a clean airtight container.

Cauliflower Kale soup

Preparation Time: 5 Minutes

Cook Time: 25 Minutes

Total Time: 30 Minutes

Yields: 15 Cups

Recipes:

- One yellow onion (diced)
- One tablespoon of Olive Oil
- One head of Cauliflower
- Ten cups of Low Sodium Vegetable Broth (2.5 L)
- Four cloves garlic (crushed)
- Three to four cups of kale (stems removed)

Directions

1. Firstly, the cauliflower head should be chopped into florets and remember to remove tough stems from kale.
2. Add heat olive oil in a big clean stockpot and then add diced onions. Cook for around five to seven minutes or until the onions turns translucent. Now, add garlic and then cook for another two minutes or until the garlic begins to fragrant.
3. Add kale, broth and cauliflower to the stockpot. Bring to a boil, lower the heat and then simmer for around ten to fifteen minutes or until the kale and cauliflower has softened.
4. With a blender or an immersion blender, blend the soup until it is smooth. Afterwards, Return to stockpot and then simmer for extra ten minutes.

5. Proceed to serve the soup hot with fresh cracked pepper.

Notes

Add a cup of coconut milk to prepare extra creamy. Bring the soup rapid boil, and then simmer for five extra minutes before serving it.

Cream of Zucchini Soup

Preparation Time: 5 Minutes

Cook Time: 20 Minutes

Total Time: 25 Minutes

Yields: 4 Servings

Recipes:

- Two cloves of garlic
- Half small onion (quartered)
- 32 ounces reduced-sodium Swanson chicken broth, or vegetable
- Black Pepper to taste
- Three medium zucchini, skin on cut in large chunks
- Kosher salt
- Two tablespoons of reduced-fat sour cream

For Topping:

- Fresh grated Parmesan cheese (if desired)

Directions

1. Firstly, you should combine onion, chicken broth, zucchini and garlic in a big clean pot over medium heat and then bring to a boil.
2. Decrease the heat and then cover. Now you should simmer until it becomes tender, around twenty minutes.
3. Take away from the heat and purée with a clean immersion blender; now add the sour cream and then purée once more until it is smooth.
4. Lastly, taste for pepper and salt and blend to taste.
5. Serve hot and enjoy.

Easy Sesame Quinoa Salad

Preparation Time: 10 Minutes

Total Time: 10 Minutes

Yields: 6 to 8 Servings

Recipes:

For The Slaw:

- Two cups cooked quinoa
- One bag shredded red cabbage (or around four cups shredded cabbage)
- 2/3 cup of thinly sliced green onions
- Two cups of shredded carrots
- Two tablespoons of sesame seeds
- Half cup of slivered or sliced almonds (toasted)

For The Sesame Honey Vinaigrette:

- Three Tablespoons rice wine vinegar
- 1/3 cup of vegetable oil (or any other preferred cooking oil)
- A pinch of Black Pepper
- One tablespoon of honey (or agave, to make this vegan)
- 1/8 teaspoon of sesame oil
- A pinch of salt
- One teaspoon of soy sauce

Directions:

To Make The Slaw:

1. Toss all recipes together until it is well combined. Serve straight away, or refrigerate in a clean sealed container for about one day.

To Make The Asian Honey Vinaigrette:

2. Whisk all recipes together until it is well combined. Then serve to enjoy.

Sweet Potato Brussels Sprout Quinoa Bowl

Yields: 4 to 6 Servings

Recipes

- One and a half cups of vegetable broth can also use chicken broth
- One cup of quinoa rinsed
- Two cloves of garlic (minced)
- One tablespoon of olive oil
- One tablespoon of fresh ginger root (diced)
- Half onion (minced)
- One cup sliced Brussels sprouts
- Two cups sweet potatoes (diced)
- 1/4 cup of sliced almonds
- Two tablespoons of dried cranberries

Directions

1. Firstly, you should place both broth and quinoa into a clean pot. Now, bring to boil over medium heat. Cover and then decrease the heat to low, now simmer for around fifteen to twenty minutes or until liquid is absorbed completely.
2. Just as the quinoa is cooking, place garlic, olive oil, ginger and onion into the big clean skillet. Cook over medium heat three to four minutes until the onions appears translucent. Add Brussels and sweet potatoes sprouts and then let cook approximately ten minutes or until they become soften.
3. Now the cooked quinoa should be added to the skillet and completely combine.
4. Take away from the heat.
5. Add almonds and cranberries and mix once more then serve to enjoy.

Curried Cauliflower

Yields: 4 Servings

Recipes:

- One teaspoon of curry Madra spice
- One cauliflower head, cut into florets.
- Half teaspoon of turmeric
- One teaspoon of cumin spice

For Roasting:

- Rock salt
- Olive oil

Directions

1. Firstly, you should heat up the oven to 180 degrees Celsius.

2. Now, add the cut cauliflower to a clean baking tray and then sprinkle over spices.
3. You should drizzle with some olive oil and rock salt. Use your hands to toss it together.
4. Roast in the oven on for twenty to twenty-five minutes or until it becomes golden and also spicy.

Italian Fennel and Orange Salad

Preparation Time: 5 Minutes

Total Time: 5 Minutes

Yields: 4 Servings

Recipes:

- One orange (peeled and sliced into thin slivers)
- One bulb fennel (rinsed and sliced into small thin strips)
- Pepper
- Salt
- Two tablespoons of olive oil

Directions

1. Firstly, you should pop the crispy fennel slices into a clean container and then gently top with the juicy orange slivers.
2. Add the olive oil and stir to combine.
3. Sprinkle with cracked black pepper & sea salt to taste.
4. Serve instantly or within one to two hours.
5. Ensure it is chilled for the crispiest texture.

Maple Sriracha Roasted Cauliflower

Preparation Time: 10 Minutes

Cook Time: 35 Minutes

Total Time: 45 Minutes

Yields: 4 Servings

Recipes:

- Two and a half tablespoons of olive oil
- One head of cauliflower (cut into bite-sized)
- Two and a half tablespoons maple syrup
- 1/4 teaspoon of pepper (or as desired)
- One and a half tablespoons of sriracha
- 1/4 teaspoon of salt (or as desired)

Directions:

1. Firstly you should heat up the oven to 425 degrees Fahrenheit.
2. Proceed to cut the cauliflower into bite-sized pieces; now move to a big clean container; put aside. In a small clean container combine sriracha, olive oil, pepper, salt and maple syrup.
3. Now gently pour the sriracha mixture over the cauliflower and mix well to combine, Ensure it is well coated in the sauce.
4. Spread the cauliflower onto a large clean baking sheet and bake for twenty minutes, stirring once at the halfway point. Increase the oven's temperature to 475 degrees Fahrenheit and then bake for extra twelve minutes, or until becomes golden brown. Serve immediately.

Baked Cinnamon Apple Chips

Preparation Time: 5 minutes

Cook Time: 3 hrs

Total Time: 3 hrs 30 minutes

Yield: 3 to 4 Servings

Recipes:

- Granulated sugar
- Three apples (I prefer Honey Crisp, Pink Lady, or Granny Smith)
- Ground cinnamon

Directions

1. Firstly you should heat up the oven to 200 degrees Fahrenheit. Carefully line two large clean baking

sheets along with clean silicone baking mats. Put aside when done.

2. Gently rinse and thinly slice the apples. Afterwards, spread the apple slices onto the clean baking pans, making one layer. Sprinkle with sugar and cinnamon.

3. Proceed to bake for one hour, you need to flip the apples over, and then bake for an extra one to one and a half hours. Put off the oven and while the apples are inside for one hour so as to let it cool (also makes it crunchy). After 3 hours in the oven, some apples may just be chewy and slightly crunchy.

4. Keep the apple chips at room temperature in a clean airtight bowl for up to one week.

Zucchini Noodles with Avocado Sauce

Preparation Time: 10 Minutes

Total Time: 10 Minutes

Yields: 2 Servings

Recipes:

- 1 1/4 cup (30grams) of basil
- One zucchini
- Four tablespoons of pine nuts
- 1/3 cup (85ml) of water
- Twelve sliced cherry tomatoes
- One avocado
- Two tablespoons of lemon juice

Directions

1. Firstly you should use a peeler or the Spiralizer to make the zucchini noodles.
2. Now you will have to blend the rest of the recipes (leaving the cherry tomatoes) in a clean blender until it is smooth.
3. Combine avocado sauce, cherry tomatoes and noodles and in a clean mixing container.
4. Zucchini noodles with avocado sauce are better if consumed while it is fresh, but you can keep them in the refrigerator up to two days.

Notes

1. You can use fresh herbs or any veggies.
2. Veggies like beet, carrots, cabbage, butternut squash etc. can be spiralized.

3. Every other nut can be used in place of the pine nuts.

Roasted Broccoli With Asiago, Garlic And Almonds

Preparation Time: 5 Minutes

Cook Time: 25 Minutes

Total Time: 25 Minutes

Yield: 4 Servings

Recipes:

- Three tablespoons of extra-virgin olive oil
- One and a half pounds of broccoli cut into small florets
- Half teaspoon of kosher salt
- Two to three cloves of garlic (sliced thin)
- One medium lemon sliced half
- ¼ teaspoon of ground black pepper

- ¼ cup of freshly grated Asiago cheese
- Three tablespoons toasted slivered almonds

Directions

1. Firstly you should heat up the oven to 425 degrees Fahrenheit and gently line a baking sheet with a clean aluminium foil.
2. In a big clean container, toss the oil, broccoli, salt, pepper and garlic. Spread equally on the pan, drizzling any surplus oil on top, and then roast in the oven for twenty to twenty-five minutes until the florets are caramelized and crispy, but still a just tender. Check the broccoli after fifteen to twenty minutes.
3. Lastly, you should squeeze the lemon over the broccoli and top with the cheese and almonds. Serve when hot.

Notes

You can add less or more olive oil, salt, lemon juice, cheese or pepper to taste. Take a peek at the broccoli after fifteen to twenty minutes; the roasting time will vary based on how small the broccoli florets are cut. If you find it hard getting Asiago cheese, Parmesan is a great alternative.

Roasted Chicken Thighs with Fennel & Lemon

Yields: 4 Servings

Recipes:

- Two small fennel bulbs
- Two pounds bone-in, skin-on chicken thighs
- One Meyer or regular lemon
- Four large cloves of garlic (minced)
- Two tablespoons of dry white wine
- Two tablespoons of olive oil
- Freshly ground black pepper.
- Cooked rice or bread, (if desired, for serving)
- One teaspoon of kosher salt

Directions

1. Firstly, you should carefully arrange a rack in the oven's centre and then heat up the oven to 425 degrees Fahrenheit. Now, place the chicken in a big clean container; put aside.
2. Now, carefully trim off the stalks and fronds of the fennel bulbs and then set aside the fronds. Cut each bulb in quarters through the root. Cut each quarter into one-inch-thick slices. Add to the container with the chicken. Add about one tablespoon of fennel fronds (minced) to the container.
3. Add garlic to the container. Finely grate the zest of the lemon into the container. Add lemon juice to the bowl. Add the white wine and oil, season with black pepper and salt, and then toss to combine.
4. Transfer the chicken mixture onto a big clean baking sheet. Carefully arrange the fennel around

the outside and the chicken pieces placed closely together in the middle. Pour any left juices from the container over the chicken.

5. Proceed to roast until the internal chicken temperature is around 160 degrees Fahrenheit and the fennel is starting to brown by the edges and also tender, approximately thirty minutes. Remove from the oven and then cover with a clean aluminium foil. Let it cool for around five to ten minutes before serving.

6. You can serve along with bread or rice if desired.

Shaved Fennel White Bean Salad With Olive Vinaigrette

Recipes:

For The Salad:

- One and a half cup of cannellini beans
- Two small or one large bulbs fennel
- Two cups of arugula
- One lemon (halved)

For The Olive Vinaigrette:

- One teaspoon of dijon mustard
- 1/4 cup of kalamata olives, pitted
- Half lemon juice
- One clove of garlic
- Three tablespoons of flat-leaf Italian parsley

- 1/4 cup of extra-virgin olive oil
- Black Pepper
- 1/4 teaspoon of fine sea salt

Directions:

1. Firstly, you would have to slice the fennel bulbs in half and then remove a tough core afterwards. Now thinly slice the fennel in rounds or half-moons with a sharp knife or a mandolin and then place in a clean salad container.
2. Now you should squeeze the lemon juice over it and then add the white beans afterwards. Using your fingertips carefully toss together lightly.
3. In a small clean blender, add all the vinaigrette recipes and then pulse until it is well combined. You can taste and to readjust if necessary.

4. Lastly, you should add vinaigrette to the wood and toss with fennel and beans. Also, add the arugula and toss again, then top with lemon zest and black pepper.

5. You can add more fennel fronds or flat-leaf parsley for more greens!

Spiralized Carrot And Fennel Salad

Preparation Time: 10 Minutes

Total Time: 10 Minutes

Yields: 4 Servings

Recipes:

- One head fennel
- Three medium-sized carrots peeled (if desired)

For The Dressing:

- One tablespoon of white wine vinegar
- Four tablespoons of extra virgin olive oil
- ¼ teaspoon of ground ginger
- Freshly ground black Pepper
- One teaspoon of honey
- Salt

- Half teaspoon chopped fresh thyme

Directions

1. Using a fork whisk all the recipes for the dressing together and put aside when you are done.
2. Now, carefully spiralize the carrots and then place in a clean container.
3. Trim the fennels (top and bottom). Remove any tough or discoloured outer leaves, then carefully cut into quarters and thinly slice. Add to the carrots to it.
4. Mix the dressing recipes once more and then pour over the salad.
5. Gently toss to coat and enjoy.

Cabbage Salad With Corn

Recipes:

- 1/2 medium of cabbage about 1 1/2 lb.
- ½ of English cucumber, sliced
- 1 cup of corn frozen and thawed or canned
- 1/3 cup of chopped dill
- 1 1/2 tbsp of vinegar
- 3 tbsp of olive oil
- 1/2 teaspoon of salt
- 1/2 teaspoon of pepper or to taste

Directions

1. Start off by very thinly slicing the cabbage. If you have one, you can use a mandolin to help you slice it.
2. In a large mixing bowl, place the sliced cabbage and add salt and pepper. Massaging the cabbage using

your hands (as if you are kneading dough). This will soften and release some juices from the cabbage so that it becomes moist.

3. Add all the remaining ingredients and mix well with each other. Just serve.

Spinach And Sun-Dried Tomato Zoodles

Recipes:

- Six zucchinis
- Two tablespoons of olive oil, divided
- ½ cup of sun-dried tomatoes in olive oil
- One tablespoon of pine nuts
- ¼ teaspoon of red pepper flakes
- One garlic clove, minced
- 2 cups of baby spinach, roughly chopped
- Juice of a half lemon
- Freshly grated Parmesan cheese
- Fresh chopped basil

Directions

1. Place the sun-dried tomatoes in a blender bowl and pulse until they are finely chopped. Transfer and set aside in a bowl.

2. Create zucchini spaghetti using a spiralizer (always read the instructions as they vary by brand - I use this spiralizer). Make use of a regular vegetable peeler to vertically peel long, thin strips of zucchini if you do not have a spiralizer. This, like fettuccini, will form more of a broader "noodle" from the zucchini.

3. Heat one tablespoon of olive oil over medium to high heat in a large skillet. Add the zucchini noodles once hot and cook for about 2 to 3 minutes, until the zucchini noodles are tender, but some crunch is still retained.

4. For about 3 minutes, let the noodles rest so that they can release all the moisture. Drain the leftover water from the pan & transfer the noodles to a colander.

5. Wipe clean, heat the skillet over medium heat & add pine nuts. Cook & stir until it is lightly toasted, about 3 minutes. Transfer and set aside in a bowl.

6. Heat the rest of the tablespoon of olive oil and add to the skillet the red flakes of pepper and garlic. Sautè for 1 minute over medium-high heat, until fragrant.

7. Add spinach and cook for about one minute, until it is almost wilted.

8. Then Add chopped sun-dried tomatoes, zoodles, & lemon juice. Stir until it is combined & heated through.

9. Sprinkle with nuts, Parmesan cheese, pine & basil.

10.   Serve and Enjoy!

Classic Potato Pancakes

Recipes:

- Four large russet potatoes
- One medium onion
- Two egg
- 1/4 cup all-purpose flour
- salt, pepper
- vegetable oil for frying

Directions

1. Peel and cube the potatoes and onion when using the food processor. Place the vegetables and process them for about 2 minutes in the food processor until the potatoes look "grated" and no lumps remain. Peel the potatoes and onion and grate when using the grater.

2. Place a fine strainer or kitchen towel with the potato mixture and try to squeeze almost all of the liquid into a clean mixing bowl.

3. Discard the fluid. After you pour the liquid out, you'll notice white powder on the bottom of the bowl. It's potato starch, and it provides the pancakes with texture, so you should keep it.

4. Return the mixture of potatoes to the bowl and add the eggs, flour, some salt, and pepper, and mix well.

5. Heat some of the vegetable oil over medium heat in a large, non-stick skillet. Add a spoonful of the potato mixture and slightly spread it out. Fry on both sides for almost 2 to 3 minutes, until the pancakes are crispy and brown.

6. On a paper towel, place the pancakes to absorb the excess oil and ENJOY!

Easy Creamy Chicken Piccata

Recipes:

- 1 Cup of Chicken Bone Broth
- 1 Lemon juiced
- ½ Cup of Coconut Cream blended before using
- ¼ Cup of Capers drained
- Lemon wedges to serve
- Freshly chopped herbs to garnish
- 1½ lbs. of Boneless, Skinless Chicken Breasts pounded to 1/2-inch thickness
- Sea salt & freshly ground black pepper
- ¼ Cup of Gluten-free Blend Flour
- 3 Tbsp of Olive Oil divided
- 4 Garlic Cloves minced
- 1 Small Onion chopped

Directions

1. On both sides, season the pounded chicken with a pinch of salt and pepper. In a clean, shallow bowl, place the flour in it.

2. Gently heat two tablespoons of oil over medium heat in a large skillet. Bring up the chicken in the flour on both sides, working with one cutlet at a time. Shake off the excess flour & add it to the saucepan.

3. Cook the chicken on each side for 4 minutes, or until it is cooked through and the coating is golden brown. Transfer to a plate the browned chicken, and set aside.

4. Lower the heat to medium-low in the same pan and add the remaining tablespoon of oil, onions, and garlic. Sauté for 2-3 minutes until the onions are softened, stirring occasionally.

5. Add the broth and lemon juice and use a silicone spatula to scrape the browned bits from the bottom of the pan. Raise the heat to a medium-high, & cook the mixture for 3 minutes, occasionally stirring, until reduced by half.
6. Stir in the cream of the coconut and the capers, and place the chicken in the sauce. Simmer over low heat for up to 3 minutes or until thoroughly heated. Season with sea salt and black pepper to taste.
7. Serve warm over sautéed cauliflower or cooked rice.

Sweet And Sour Cucumber Noodles

Recipes:

- 3 teaspoons of fresh lemon or lime juice
- 3 TBSP of extra virgin olive oil
- 2 TBSP of white vinegar
- 1/4 tsp of salt plus extra, to taste
- 1/8 tsp of dill (fresh or dried)
- 1/8 tsp of garlic powder
- 1/2 tsp of fresh minced garlic
- 1/4-1/2 cup of fresh chopped cilantro plus extra to garnish
- 2 TBSP of honey
- 2 TBSP of rice vinegar
- One big English cucumber
- Toasted sesame seeds & chia seeds for topping

Directions

1. Whisk everything together but the last three recipes and pour over the noodles.
2. To soak up all the yummy dressing or pop it in the fridge for later, let them sit at room temperature.
3. Whisk the honey and rice vinegar together before serving and drizzle heartfully over the noodles.
4. Garnish with a sprinkle of cilantro or chopped green onion with toasted sesame seeds and/or chia seeds.
5. Crushed peanuts or cashews are also excellent! Based on what you have available as well as what you prefer taste/topping-wise, it is ridiculously simple to customize! Grab an English giant cucumber, a veggie peeler/spiral slicer, and go nuts!
6. Serve for maximum flavor at room temperature.

Roasted Broccoli Quinoa Salad

Recipes:

- 1 cup dry quinoa

- 2 cups water (or veggie broth)

- ½ pound broccoli, cut into florets

- One sweet potato, chopped into ¼ – ½ inch chunks

- One can (15 oz) chickpeas

- One bunch laccinto kale, roughly chopped

- olive oil, as needed

- 1/3 cup fresh parsley

- 3 Tablespoons feta cheese

- juice from one lemon

- 1/2 Tablespoon apple cider vinegar

- Two teaspoons maple syrup

- 3 Tablespoons olive oil

- salt and ground pepper, to taste

- crushed red pepper, to taste (optional)

Directions

1. Then bring the quinoa & water to a boil in a clean medium saucepan. Cover, reduce the heat to low, & simmer until the quinoa is tender or for 15 minutes. Remove from the heat & all to stand, covered, for up to 5 minutes. Use a fork to remove the lid and the fluff. To a large bowl, transfer the quinoa.

2. To the quinoa, add roasted broccoli, spinach, and green onion. Drizzle it with fresh lemon juice & olive oil. Stir gently. Add the feta cheese, chopped pistachios, and season with salt and black pepper to taste. Just serve.

Honey Garlic Roasted Carrots

Recipes:

- 2 pounds of carrots cut into 3-inch pieces
- 1/2 cup of butter
- 2 tbsp of honey
- Four garlic cloves minced
- 1/2 tsp of salt
- 1/4 tsp of fresh ground pepper
- Freshly parsley

Directions

1. Preheat the oven to 425°C
2. Melt the butter in an oven-proof skillet. Add in honey & garlic and whisk until combined.
3. Add in the carrots and coat with a toss.
4. Bake in the oven until the carrots are fork-tender or for 25 minutes.

5. Optional- To caramelize the carrots a bit, broil for 3-4 minutes.

6. Sprinkle with parsley that has been chopped.

Kale Salad

Recipes:

- 1 lb. of kale
- One large semi-sweet apple
- 1/3 cup of roasted almonds

Dressing Ingredients:

- 3 tbsp. of extra virgin olive oil
- 2 tbsp. of freshly squeezed lemon juice
- One garlic clove
- A half teaspoon of salt

Directions

1. Remove the kale stalks and discard them. Roll the kale into a bunch and thinly slice the leaves.

2. In a clean large mixing bowl, gently place the kale leaves. Add the salt & massage the leaves until the kale starts to soften plus wilt, about 2-3 minutes.
3. Add the kale with the olive oil, lemon juice, and garlic. Stir thoroughly and set aside.
4. Peel the apple and core it. Dice it into small pieces & add them to the salad. Stir well, everything.
5. In a serving bowl, transfer the salad and sprinkle the nuts on top. Just serve.

Garlic Herb Roasted Potatoes Carrots And Green Beans

Recipes:

- 1 1/4 pounds of baby red potatoes (halved and larger ones quartered)
- 1 pound of medium carrots (scrubbed clean, cut into 2-inch pieces and thicker portions halved)
- Three tablespoons of olive oil (divided)
- One tablespoon of fresh thyme (minced)
- One tablespoon of fresh rosemary (minced)
- Salt
- freshly ground black pepper
- 12 ounces of green beans (ends trimmed, halved)
- 1 1/2 tablespoons of minced garlic (4 cloves)

Directions

1. Preheat the oven to 400°C. Toss potatoes, carrots with 2 1/2 tablespoons olive oil, thyme, rosemary in a large bowl & season with salt & pepper to taste. On a rimmed 18 by 13-inch baking clean sheet, spread. Roast for up to 20 minutes in a preheated oven.

2. In a bowl, combine the green beans with the remaining 1/2 Tbsp of olive oil and lightly season with salt. Add other veggies to the baking sheet, add garlic and toss everything and spread it into an even layer. Return to the oven & roast for up to 20 minutes until all the veggies are tender and slightly browned. Serve it hot.

Roasted Cauliflower Steaks

Recipes:

- Two heads of cauliflower
- One teaspoon of kosher salt
- ½ teaspoon of black pepper
- ½ teaspoon of garlic powder
- ½ teaspoon of paprika
- ¼ cup of olive oil
- One teaspoon of chopped parsley

Directions

1. Adjust the oven rack to the third position below. Preheat to 260oC (500oF)
2. Remove the green outer leaves from the cauliflower head & trim the stem.
3. Gently cut the cauliflower in half lengthwise through the center using a large knife.

4. From each half, cut a one and half-inch-thick steak. Carefully cut one more steak from each of the cut sides of the head is large.
5. Repeat with the other cauliflower head process. Trim any florets which are not linked to the stem. About 4 to 8 pieces in total should be there.
6. On a rimmed baking sheet, put the cauliflower steaks.
7. Mix the salt, pepper, garlic powder, and paprika together in a small bowl.
8. Drizzle each side of each cauliflower steak with olive oil.
9. Sprinkle the seasoning mixture evenly, about 1/4 teaspoon per side, on both sides of the cauliflower steaks.
10. Close well the baking sheet tightly with a clean foil & bake for 5 minutes.

11. Take the cauliflower off the foil and roast for 10 minutes.
12. Flip the cauliflower steak gently and roast until both sides form a golden-brown crust, about 7 to 8 mins.
13. Move to a serving dish & garnish with par filling.

Hot Turkey And Cheese Party Rolls

Recipes:

- 1 Stick of Butter Melted (½ cup)
- One 8 ounces tube of Crescent Roll Dough
- 12 to 16 Slices of Turkey (Deli Sliced)
- 12 to 14 slices of Colby Jack Cheese
- ¼ teaspoon of Garlic Powder
- 2 Tbsp. of Chopped Parsley
- 1 tsp. of Poppy Seed

Directions

1. Roll out Crescent Roll Dough & press the diagonal seam together into four rectangle shapes.
2. Put 3-4 slices of turkey and cheese on each rectangle.

3. Roll each rectangle up (roll from one short side to the next short side) and gently press the seam together (You will have four rolls at this point).
4. For a total of 12 rolls, slice each roll into three pieces.
5. Spray cooking spray on a 9/13 baking dish
6. Place rolls in a baking pan with 9/13
7. Combine the butter, garlic powder, and parsley in a small bowl.
8. Crescent Rolls Brush over and Sprinkle with Poppy Seed
9. Bake for up to 15 minutes, at 350 degrees, until it just starts to turn brown.

Roasted Broccoli Fennel Soup

Preparation Time: 5 Minutes

Cook time: 30 Minutes

Total time: 35 Minutes

Yields: 4 Servings

Recipes:

- Two cups of fennel (chopped into wedges)
- Four cups of broccoli florets
- Five cloves of garlic (minced)
- Two tablespoons of olive oil (divided)
- Two cups curly kale (ribs removed)
- One medium onion (chopped)
- Three cups filtered water
- Black Pepper

- Half cup of raw cashews
- Three big handfuls of baby kale
- Two tablespoons of lemon juice
- Sea salt

Directions

1. Firstly, you should heat up the oven to 400 degrees Fahrenheit, and gently line a baking sheet with a clean parchment paper.
2. Spread fennel and broccoli equally on the prepared clean baking sheet, drizzle with one tablespoon of olive oil and then roast for twenty minutes, turning fennel and broccoli after ten minutes.
3. In the meantime, in a big clean saucepot over medium to low heat, add minced garlic and the left tablespoon of olive oil and sweat for three minutes. Add the onion and sweat for another five minutes.

As soon as the fennel and broccoli are done roasting, add them to the saucepan and then stir thoroughly once again.

4. Then add in the cashews, kale, lemon juice, water and kale, and season with pepper and salt. Simmer the mixture for five minutes, Take away from heat and then blend until it is smooth.
5. Serve when the soup is warm, top with the dukkah.

Note

1. Use less water (two cups) if you want to make this without the cashews.
2. Other greens such as collards and spinach can be used in place baby kale.
3. You can store in a clean airtight container in the refrigerator for about three days if prepared earlier.

Leek, Sweet Potato and Rosemary Soup

Preparation Time: 20 Minutes

Cook Time: 30 Minutes

Total Time: 50 Minutes

Yields: 4 Servings

Recipes:

- Two leeks finely diced
- Low-calorie cooking spray
- Four large sweet potatoes (peeled and chopped)
- One teaspoon of fresh rosemary finely chopped.
- Two cloves of garlic crushed.
- Freshly ground pepper
- Chicken stock (1 L)
- A sprinkling of rosemary (for garnish)

- Salt

Directions

1. Using a cooking spray, gently spray the bottom of a big clean saucepan around five times. Turn on heat at high temperature; as soon as the oil begins to bubble turn down the heat to a medium temperature.
2. Sauté the garlic and leeks for two to three minutes, continually stirring to avoid burning.
3. Add the rosemary and chopped potatoes and then stir around the pan for one minute or thereabout.
4. Add the chicken stock and simmer for roughly twenty to twenty-five minutes until it is soft.
5. With a clean stick blender or in a clean food processor, puree the soup to a thick consistency.
6. Take back to the pan and then season to taste.

7. Garnish with a sprinkling of rosemary on top before serving.

Notes

You can store in a freezer.

Creamy Asparagus and Leek Soup

Preparation Time: 10 Minutes

Cook time: 15 Minutes

Total Time: 25 Minutes

Yields: 7 Servings

Recipes:

- Two leeks (chopped)
- Two bunches of asparagus (chopped)
- Two tablespoons of coconut oil
- One teaspoon of Pepper
- Four cloves of garlic
- One can of full-fat coconut milk.
- Two cups of vegetable broth (gluten-free)

Directions

1. In a big clean soup pan, sautée the leeks, asparagus, pepper, coconut oil and garlic over medium to high heat for five to seven minutes, until vegetables become tender.
2. Move the cooked vegetables to a clean blender, add one can of coconut milk and hot vegetable stock. Blend at high speed for three to five minutes until it gets smooth and also creamy.
3. Serve to enjoy.

Wild Salmon With Braised Vegetables

Yields: 4 Servings

Recipes:

- Stone salt
- Four wild salmon pieces (150grams each)
- One tablespoon of coconut oil
- Dill
- A pinch of lemon zest

For The Vegetables:

- 200grams of Chervil root
- 200grams of parsley root
- Stone salt
- One tablespoon of olive oil
- Dried oregano
- Nutmeg

For The Dill Potato Base Sauce:

- Vegetable broth or 500ml water
- 200grams of peeled potatoes (wash and peel)
- One tablespoon of dill
- Cream (to taste)
- Nutmeg
- Stone salt

Directions

1. Fill a clean saucepan with vegetable broth or the water, now add in the potatoes and then boil until it is soft. Puree the boiled potatoes with the liquid using a blender jug or hand blender. Add water or broth just as required to give the sauce a creamy consistency. Add the dill and froth up with the cream. Add nutmeg and stone salt to taste.

2. Now you should heat up the oven to 150 degrees Celsius. Gently rinse and peel the chervil roots and parsley root. Marinate with nutmeg, salt, oregano and olive oil. Put the vegetables in a clean roasting tin, add water (125ml) and then braise in the oven for roughly thirty minutes.

3. Just before the vegetables are done, season the salmon with lemon zest, dill and salt. Carefully fry the salmon with the skin-side down in a clean frying pan in some coconut oil. Place in the oven along with the vegetables for about five to seven minutes until it is totally cooked.

4. Add the vegetables on a dish and then add the sauce. Take out the cooked salmon from the oven and top on the vegetables.

5. Enjoy.

Grilled Beet and Fennel Salad

Preparation Time: 10 Minutes

Cook Time: 20 Minutes

Total Time: 30 Minutes

Yields: 4 Servings

Recipes:

- One orange zest
- One cup of plain plant-based yoghurt or Greek yoghurt or plain coconut yoghurt
- One pinch of salt
- Half teaspoon of cumin
- Two tablespoons of olive oil
- 1/4 teaspoon of Black Pepper
- Two fennel bulbs trimmed and cut into half-inch thick slices

- Four to five beets steamed, peeled and cut into half-inch rounds
- 1/4 cup of sprouted lentils
- Black lava salt (if desired)
- Fennel fronds

Directions

1. In a small clean container, stir together orange zest, coconut yoghurt, pepper, salt and cumin. Put aside.
2. Now heat up a clean grill pan over medium to high heat. Gently brush with the oil and then grill beet and fennel slices, do it in batches, for approximately two to three minutes for each side. Take away from the heat and then let to it cool slightly.
3. Carefully spread a thin layer of yoghurt onto a platter. Top with grilled beets, sprouted lentils and grilled fennel.

4. Drizzle with olive oil and garnish with fennel fronds and black lava salt.

Cabbage, Cucumber and Fennel Salad with Dill

Total Time: 1 hour 30 Minutes

Yields: 10 Servings

Recipes:

- One medium sweet onion (very thinly sliced on a mandolin)
- 1¼ pounds of Savoy cabbage (very thinly sliced on a mandoline (six cups))
- Ice water
- One and a half pounds fennel bulbs (halved, cored & very thinly shaved on a mandolin)
- Kosher salt
- One seedless cucumber (halved lengthwise & sliced crosswise 1/8-inch thick)

- Two tablespoons white wine vinegar
- One cup of crème fraîche
- Three tablespoons poppy seeds
- Half cup chopped dill

Directions

1. Put the onion, fennel and cabbage in three different containers and add some ice water let it cover; leave for thirty minutes.
2. Now gently drain the vegetables and then spin dry using a clean salad spinner. In a different clean bowl, toss the cucumbers with two teaspoons of salt and then add some ice water, let it cover. Leave for thirty minutes, then drain once more and then pat dry.
3. In a very big clean container, whisk the crème fraîche with the vinegar until it is firm. Add the

poppy seeds and dill and season with salt. Fold in the onion, cabbage, cucumber and fennel and serve immediately.

Corn Soup with Lemongrass

Recipes:

- Chopped fresh mint (as desired)
- 150grams of corn
- 150ml of cream substitute sea salt /soup seasoning rice syrup or whipped cream
- 200ml of vegetable stock
- Lemongrass

Directions

1. Bring the vegetables and corn to a boil, cut the lemongrass. Add the lemongrass to the soup and then simmer for around fifty minutes.
2. Take out the lemongrass and then puree the soup and pass through a strainer afterwards.
3. Add the recipes left and puree once more.

4. Lastly, add fresh mint and serve to enjoy.

Note

For Main Dish:

1. Add pikeperch filet, carefully fry the fish in some coconut oil or olive oil then add in soup before serving.
2. Serve to enjoy!

Red Beet Cake

Recipes:

- 100grams of whole-grain spelt flour
- 100grams of honey
- 200grams of red beets (rinsed, peeled and finely grated)
- Five eggs
- 200grams of freshly ground almonds

Directions

1. Firstly separate the egg whites and yolks.
2. Whisk the egg yolks and the honey. Gently blend in the almonds, flour and red beets, then thoroughly stir.
3. Beat the eggs white until it is firm, then gently fold into the mixture.

4. Gently pour the prepared dough into a greased clean baking tray.
5. Lastly, you should heat up the oven at 170 degrees Celsius for about 1 hour until it appears golden brown.
6. Then take out of the oven and serve to enjoy.

Rack of Lamb with Polenta

Recipes:

- 180ml of water
- 120grams of polenta (refine with cream and rub with garlic)
- Rosemary
- 500grams of a rack of lamb
- Sea salt
- 10grams of Aslan, coconut oil or butter

Directions

1. Firstly, you will have to season rack of lamb in Aslan, coconut oil or butter then wrap in a clean aluminium foil and take to the oven to roast at 180 degrees Celsius for approximately ten minutes until it is ready.

2. Ensure the meat is pink inside and any juice discharge should be combined with butter when preparing the sauce.
3. Add polenta in water with butter or Aslan then cook, let it cool for some minutes.
4. Add seasonal herbs to add flavour, form small patties and then fry until gets crispy with some coconut oil or butter.
5. Serve to enjoy.

Note

You can also bake rack of lamb in polenta crust or goat cheese.

Conclusion

This Essential Mayr Diet Cookbook would serve as a guide to weight loss and will give you amazing ideas for delicious recipes

The recipes are adequate for all cooking skill levels and are great to prepare with the families.

Get lean and stay healthy.

Enjoy!

Made in United States
Cleveland, OH
11 August 2025